VASCULAR ACCESS CATHETER MATERIALS AND EVOLUTION

VASCULAR ACCESS CATHETER MATERIALS AND EVOLUTION

Joseph D. Giusto

Copyright © 2014 by Joseph D. Giusto.

ISBN: Softcover   978-1-4990-3980-1
             eBook   978-1-4990-3979-5

All rights reserved. No part of this book may be reproduced or transmitted in any form or by any means, electronic or mechanical, including photocopying, recording, or by any information storage and retrieval system, without permission in writing from the copyright owner.

Any people depicted in stock imagery provided by Thinkstock are models, and such images are being used for illustrative purposes only.
Certain stock imagery © Thinkstock.

This book was printed in the United States of America.

Rev. date: 06/18/2014

To order additional copies of this book, contact:
Xlibris LLC
1-888-795-4274
www.Xlibris.com
Orders@Xlibris.com
552659

CONTENTS

I. Introduction 7
II. The Evolution of the Vascular Catheter 9
    a. Natural Rubber 13
    b. Synthetic Rubber 15
    c. Thermoplastic Rubbers 16
    d. Polyurethanes 17
    e. Polyvinylchloride (PVC) 20
    f. Silicone Rubber 22
    g. Dacron Felt Cuffs: as Anchors and as
       Infection Barriers 24
    h. Venous Access Port 25
    i. Silicone Rubber Cross-Linking Systems 26
III. Silicone Rubber Atrial Catheters – Compared 27
    a. Tunneled External CVC's – Silicone
       Large Bore Catheters 27
IV. Plastics – Other 29
    a. Polyethylene 29
    b. Teflon 30
    c. Nylon 30
V. Horizons for VAD Materials 31
VI. References 33

INTRODUCTION

This chapter will hopefully serve to give the reader an understanding of the early materials used as catheters. Those devices, generally first used urologically, eventually expanded to vascular applications.

The gradual evolution from the crudest drain tubes, rigid in nature, to the current state where soft, flexible and much more biologically compatible elastomerics are employed, is discussed here.

Just as important were those trail blazing, courageous and daring early clinical investigators. Some of these people allowed themselves to be used for the first known human heart catheterization experiments. The material used was that available in the period, namely natural rubber catheters.

Besides rubber, other materials considered for vascular access and discussed are synthetic rubber, thermoplastic elastomers, polyurethanes, polyvinylchloride (PVC) and silicone rubber.

Also described in this review are the cuffs, serving the dual purpose of anchoring the catheter and as an infection barrier, subcutaneous port materials and the lesser used catheter plastics such as polyethylene, Teflon and Nylon.

Where we are going in this field of materials for vascular access is addressed. The forecasted direction is current materials improvements either through modifications of their chemistries and/or coatings. Catheter design changes in physical appearance, allowing the stiffer materials which are otherwise compatible, to be more safely placed and to remain in place more safely, is another possibility.

THE EVOLUTION OF THE VASCULAR CATHETER

If documentation were available from the very first time a catheter was used it would most likely indicate that the tube was a hollowed out reed or some such natural material. Also, it probably would describe its use as a tool in urology needs.

A catheter is defined as any of various tubular medical devices whose design is for insertion into body canals, vessels, passageways or cavities, to allow injection or withdrawal of fluids or other substances or to maintain the patency of a passageway.

Thus, it is the imagination, solely, that can limit what could be used as a catheter, and, of course, the consequences of choice and body part affected.

A few of the rigid catheter materials include glass or metal. The latter instruments consisted of bronze, unearthed in Pompei excavations and from that period to the early 1700's, silver copper, brass, wax and even horn had been used. In the 1840's, silver plated and steel catheters were used. The problem with these urinary catheters was rigidity. The challenge for more flexibility was offered by Solingen's spiral catheter (1706) and in 1871 by Lewis Sayre of New Jersey with his vertebrate silver catheter. Independently, T.H. Squire of Elmira, New York, had a remarkably similar solution.[1]

Better as they were, bendable metal was not the answer to patient comfort. In 1877, the J. Elwood Lee Company, Conshohoken, Pennsylvania produced the first of today's woven textile catheter with a few layers of flexible varnish.[2]

The French were not standing still and had their own versions of flexible catheters. In fact, at the end of the nineteenth century, French urologist J. J. Cazenave used as a starting material, a cylinder of ivory. After a series of chemical processing it was indeed transformed into a softened draining tube.[3]

The advent of vulcanized rubber was to change this scene. Failures of early natural rubber catheters, led to the manufacture, for a short period, of catheters of "mineralized India Rubber".[4]

A few other references note that other metals were used. For instance, in an emergency situation, a distended bladder of a spinal injured boy was relieved by a Dr. William Shaw of Edgefield District, South Carolina, using a bar of lead, hammered thin, rolled into a knitting needle to form a tube and introducing this into the victim.[5]

Other catheter materials were not previously mentioned are plaster[6], platinum or other non-corroding metal[7], and "a gum catheter...about 20 years before"[8].

The first indication of angioaccess is that of Richard Lower's experiments involving two dogs linked via a series of quills from the carotid artery of one dog ot the jugular vein of another.[9] In 1730, vascular monitoring was performed by a Stephan Hales, who placed a hollow brass rod into a horse's carotid artery.[10]

Cardiac catheterization development to a sophisticated level, in animal studies in the 1840's, is credited to a rather profound French physiologist, Claude Bernard.[11]

In a letter to the Lancet, a Gerald R. Graham, tells of Claude Bernard's experiments that the latter published in detail in 1855. The withdrawal of blood from the right heart of a living dog was through a metal catheter.[12]

Another claim to original cardiac catheterization was made by a Professor Arrigo Montanari, Lecci, Italy. He carried this technique from living dogs to human cadavers. The results were apparently published in *Sperimental* in January 1929.[13]

The 1956 Nobel Prize for Medicine was awarded to one German and two American physicians for cardiac catheterization.

The German was Werner Forssman, whose experiments date back to 1929, and, in fact, the spectacular self experiment was published by him on November 5, 1929.[14]

However, in a letter to *JAMA*, a Frederick E. Ems, MD, claims that Fritz Bleichroeder, Chief Resident of the medical department of the Municipal Hospital Gitschienerstrasse in Berlin, Germany, performed a catheterization of the heart in 1908. It was after Bleichroeder's numerous successful dog experiments that he, Fritz Bleichroeder, catheterized the heart of a laboratory assistant, Joseph Portmann, using a ureteral catheter.[15]

In a confirmation of the above, F. Bleichroeder, is again credited with the procedure of heart catheterization of a human, and, in 1912, he had himself catheterized. A flexible rubber catheter was used in both dogs and man to (1) reach into his arm and thigh veins and finally into the vena cava, and, (2) into veins and arteries of patients.[16]

W. Forssman's first human experiments were on cadavers. Using this confidence, he had an assistant perform the final attempt of catheterization on himself. The catheter used was a Number 4 Charriere ureteral catheter, stored in sterile olive oil. However, the experiment was aborted after inserting 34 cm into the cephalic vein. Only a week later, Forssman did it all by himself, performing venesection on his left arm under local anesthesia, inserting 65 cm of the catheter until it reached his right atrium and the important step of taking x-rays along the catheter route to prove its final placement, radiographic evidence.[17]

Because Forssman injected a radiopaque substance into the catheter and thus into his heart, we may consider him the pioneer of angiocardiography.

A Dr. P.L. Farinas, a pioneer in the field of femoral catheterization for retrograde aortography, used a natural rubber ureteral catheter, inserted through a trocar.[18]

Also, in 1941, based on the successes of those above and the confidence from their own animal experiments, Andre Cournand, H.A. Ranges and Dickinson W. Richards, clinical investigators, introduced catheters into the right heart of man and left in place for approximately one hour. Hemodynamics, i.e. pressures, blood gases, and cardiac output, were measured, and, by 1945, hundreds of such cardiac catheterization s had been performed without mishap.[19]

It has been the collective contributions of each of these courageous people to significantly advance the technique of vascular access.

One of the essential factors for progress is the improvement of catheter designs, i.e. catheter materials.

Natural Rubber

The earliest of vascular access catheters were of natural rubber. In fact, it was a rubber ureteral catheter that Werner Forssman used on himself (1929)[20] and by Fritz Bleichroeder (1912)[21] as well.

Rubber use is documented by the Europeans who first explored South and Central America in the early 1800's, the indigenous source of natural rubber. The magic of the "weeping wood", called "cachuc" by the natives and "caucho" by the Spaniards, was so named because when the bark of a particular tree (Hevea Brasiliensia), from the jungles of the rain forests was punctured, a milky fluid, i.e. latex, flowed out.

Joseph Priestley gave it the simple name "rubber" in 1770, when he found that the solidified material could rub out pencil marks.

When dried, the rubber was flexible, elastic, tough, fairly impermeable to air and even waterproof. Yet, it had major problems since it became stiff and cracked in cold weather and soft and sticky in hot weather.

In an accidental observation, Charles Goodyear in 1839, noted a dramatic change occurring when rubber was heated with sulfur present. Incorporating sulfur into soft rubber by a kneading process, Goodyear in the United States and Hancock in England, independently and at approximately the same time, laid the foundation for what was to be the gigantic rubber industry.

The period of 1920-1940 was characterized by tremendous strides in methods of production of natural and synthetic rubbers and equally important, a vast quality improvement.

Age, heat, abrasion and oxidation resistors (antioxidants), faster vulcanizing enhancers (accelerators) and strengthening compounding ingredients (reinforcing agents) all helped mushroom the practicality of rubber.

The organic accelerators also made possible the development of articles directly from latex by the dipping process.

"Dry rubber", formed into bales after field latex is coagulated, usually with formic acid, compressed, sheeted and dried, needs to be softened or masticated on open mills or in internal mixers to allow it to accept compounding ingredients. These ingredients generally include plasticizer/lubricant, retarder, accelerator, antioxidant, activator, cure agents (sulfur, sulfur bearing, metal oxides, peroxides) colorants and fillers, either reinforcing or non-reinforcing.

From this list, one can easily see that there is much that can potentially bleed, bloom or even if surface held, may affect human physiology.

The forming process, remaining with our subject catheters, is an extrusion of tubing shapes, with either single or multiple lumens. Molding parts is via compression, transfer, or injection molding.

Natural rubber *latex* has been the source of recent concerns because of allergic contact dermatitis including intraoperative anaphylaxis.[22]

Synthetic Rubber

War had its influence on the synthetic rubber development. The First World War, with the blockade of Germany, brought about that country's making small amounts of methyl rubber.

By the late 1920's, Germany laid the ground work for its Buna-S, a styrene-butadiene rubber (1933) and Buna-N, Nitrile-butadiene rubber (1936).

DuPont's polychloroprene (Neoprene) (1931) and Thiokol's polysulfide rubber (1927) was followed by Exxon's butyl rubber (1940). All the above are used in environments that preclude the use of natural rubber.[23]

All these discoveries, though called "synthetics" are not remotely close to the chemical analog of natural rubber. It was in 1953-1954 that two independently laboring scientists, Ziegler (Switzerland) and Natta (Italy) discovered a very new and exciting means of controlling the geometry of polymer molecules, via a new catalyst systems, all this while working on a true synthetic version of natural rubber, i.e. cis-polyisoprene.

Their labors offered the fruits of linear, crystalline polyethylene and polypropylene. It also caused the first cis-polyisoprene rubber to become fact in 1954.[24]

The vulcanized rubbers, because of problems with biocompatibility in chronic vascular use, never were strong contenders in this field.

Thermoplastic Rubbers

As the term thermoplastic indicates, these are a group of materials possessing elastic properties but without the need of vulcanizing or cross-linking.

The 1960 and 1970's saw a proliferation of these, including Shell's Kraton™ (1965), DuPont's Hytrel™ (copolyether ester copolymer) and Uniroyal's TPR™, a blend of ethylene-propylene diene terpolymer (EDPM) with polypropylene.

Polyurethane, a name ascribed to a rather heterogeneous 58 year old (1937) family of polymers, comprise an assortment of products from the very soft to rigid. We are interested in the implantable grade polyurethanes, and more specifically, the thermoplastic polyurethane elastomers. This class of materials meets the "elastomer" definition since it can be stretched to a reasonable point, returns again to a reasonably close original length and is very strong, all great physical properties, not unlike cured natural rubber.[25]

Polyurethanes

Some of the biomedical grades of polyurethanes elastomers are listed in Table 1.[26] A number of these have been withdrawn from the market. Chief among them are Biomer™, one of the most widely researched polyurethanes in biomedical use and those Pellethanes used in cardiac prosthetic devices and other long term implants.[27]

Name	Supplier	Description
Angioflex	Abiomed	Silicone: Urethane Copolymer
Biomer	Ethicon	Aromatic co(polyetherurea)
Cardiothane	Kontron	Silicone: Urethane Copolymer
Chrono Flex	Poly Medics	Aliphatic Non-ether
Corplex	Corvita	Silicone Covalently Bonded to Urethane
Hemothane	3M: Sarns Division	Similar to Biomer
Mitrathane	Poly Medica	Similar to Biomer
Pellethane	Dow Chemical	Aromatic Ether-Based
Surethane	Thermedics	Purified Lycra (Aromatic Ether Polyurethane)
Tecoflex	Thermedics	Aliphatic Ether-Based

Table 1

The strength of this material, plus good general blood compatibility, made it a likely candidate for cardiac prostheses. A permanent implant or total support of circulation has eluded clinicians but systems development continues.[28]

Polyurethanes generally have a tensile strength of greater than 3,000 psi and a hardness range of 75 Shore A to 75 Shore D. Compared to silicone rubber hardness range of 10 Shore A to 80 Shore A, it is very much a harder, stiffer material overall.

Abrasion resistance and radiation resistance are relatively good compared to other elastomers.

Major expenditures of resources have been allocated to study and overcome the phenomenon of blood-surface interaction with a foreign material. Polyurethanes are no exception and though it is an inherently hydrophilic material, coating to make the surface less able to absorb protein should make it less thrombogenic. Albumin, attached to polyurethanes, has improved blood compatibility.[29]

The advantages of polyurethane are the points already stated, superior abrasion resistance, hemocompatibility, outstanding mechanical properties, plus extremely great flex endurance, and the ability to be chemically altered to offer flexible, semi-rigid or rigid versions.[30]

The other side of the coin, the disadvantages, list oxidation, degradation via chain scission, environmental stress cracking (ESC), calcification and hydrolysis.[31]

These describe the ether-based polyurethanes. A new ether-free polyurethane has arrived on the scene and early testing indicated that not only did this material exhibit very good physical properties, tensile strength over 5,000 psi and elongation of nearly 600%, but animal testing showed remarkable degradation-free test pieces (no ESC).[32]

The ether-free polyurethane is a Poly Medica Industries product named Chrono Flex™ AL-80A urethane. The hypothesis is that since it contains no ether linkages, they are not acceptable to degradation from the body's enzymes or oxidants.[33]

In addition to polyurethane material being used alone in a vascular access catheter, it has been utilized as a coating, especially for woven catheters.

A radiopaque urethane coated catheter over a braided base is described as follows. The textile braid may consist of knitted or woven nylon, Dacron™, or Orlon™. The polyurethane coating may be sprayed or dipped applied and air dried or baked. Because cardiac catheters should be radiopaque, to follow the path in the body via fluoroscope, metal powders such as tin, lead and bismuth have been added to the fluid urethane.[34]

An early version of braided catheters used an oleoresin instead of a polyurethane coating. These coatings could be called a varnish or alkyd resin finish. Hand braided silk was used prior to 1800, with cotton replacing silk after that. France, Italy and Germany only made these woven catheters up to 1939. By 1941, much of the hand labor was eliminated as production spread to the United States.[35]

Polyurethane catheters are used in peripherally placed ports, as alternatives to chest wall ports or to long term external central lines.

A newly developed peripherally implanted port, Bard Cath-Link 20™ designed for access with a standard over-the-needle system, for therapies including hyperalimentation and blood products has been described in a paper.[36]

Non-port, peripherally inserted central venous catheters (PICC's) are sometimes used with infusion pumps, especially for total parenteral nutrition (TPN). Other types of therapy are antibiotics, chemotherapy, pain management, hydration and blood products.

Percutaneous, non-tunneled, central lines are another group that uses, most usually, polyurethane or silicone materials. Natural rubber was first used, followed by polyethylene, Teflon and polyvinylchloride (PVC).[37]

Interesting is a 1983 article that reaches the conclusion that a *soft* polyurethane and a *soft* polyvinylchloride venous catheter have quite similar thrombogenicity.[38]

Polyvinylchloride (PVC)

PVC, or Vinyl, must be compounded with plasticizers to make it flexible and elastomeric. Along with a plasticizer, a stabilizer, antioxidant, and, perhaps, a colorant, are usually incorporated into the PVC formulation.

In a biomedical application, the additives must not be leachable, or even to not migrate.

Certainly, this was not possible with early PVC catheters (1950's). With the Deseret Intracath, a silicone-coated polyvinyl 8-inch catheter, dramatic improvement regarding local reaction versus a PVC tubing that was not coated, was shown when used on patients.[39]

PVC is a relatively low cost material, easily formed, especially by extrusion and being thermoplastic, pulled down to correct dimensions with little difficulty.

The use of this very versatile plastic for healthcare products began in 1949, when endotracheal tubes were shaped over a copper tubing mandrel, with heat supplied by boiling water.[40]

Early pacemaker catheters were constructed of a soft PVC with a thin walled (natural rubber) latex balloon situated between the two stainless steel pacing electrodes at the catheter tip.[41] Another PVC item of this period was a tapered 28FR flexible radiopaque tube for a left heart bypass during patient cardiogenic shock.[42]

Earlier yet, we had a translucent vinyl plastic Lillehei-Warden venous circuit and cardiovascular catheter (C.R. Bard, 1958).

The development of a flow-directed catheter in 1970, by Swan and Ganz, simplified the measurement of right ventricular, pulmonary artery and wedge pressures.[43] It was described as a dual lumen, polyvinylchloride catheter, 100cm in length and an outside diameter of 1.6mm, and balloon-tipped.[44] By 1989, it had four lumens, 110cm long, heparin-coated, with a thermistor at the distal end.[45]

Today, a series of PVC/polyurethane graft polymers, with lower extractability are available for medical applications.[46]

PVC, as is the case for natural rubber, is not normally considered for devices intended for long term implantation.

A chronology of the evolution of modern day PVC may be useful in a better understanding of this material.[47]

1835 Regnault prepared vinyl chloride
1872 Baumann reported polymerization of vinyl chloride
1912 Klatte synthesized vinyl chloride
1912 Ostromislenski patented polymerization of vinyl chloride
1930 Semon plasticized PVC
1940 Production of PVC in United Kingdom

The first commercial use of PVC was in 1928, under the name Vinylite™.[48]

Silicone Rubber

Silicone rubber, the industry standard, is so important to the field of vascular access that it behooves us to follow its birth.

Silicon, the element building block of the rubber "silicone", was isolated in 1824 by Johann Berzelius. In 1863, Friedrich Wohler suggested it to be an analogy to carbon compounds. However, it was the work of Professor F.S. Kippinger, England that earned him the title of Father of Organosilicon Chemistry. In the period of 1899 to 1944, he published more than 50 papers, and eventually offering proof of that analogy between carbon and silicon.[49]

It was Kipping who coined the term "silicone" for a silicon compound which he thought was like a ketone in its structure.[50]

The Dow Corning Corporation was formed in 1943 and by 1944, the first materials produced were silicone fluids for the war efforts. In 1945, both Dow Corning and the General Electric Company announced the development of a silicone rubber.

Generally, silicones are usually referred to as polydimethlysiloxanes, which are in fluid form, and become more viscous with increasing molecular weight. Silicone rubber thus consists of a silicone fluid, a reinforcing filler and a vulcanizing agent. Or course, this is simplified but one can readily see how few ingredients are necessary to make it a viable medical product. The less compounding ingredients, the less the chance of potential complications.

By chance, it was discovered very early in the history of silicones, that when coated on glass, making it non-wetting to water, the clotting time of blood was prolonged when in this particular glassware.

The theory was that since it took longer for blood to clot when in contact with silicone than for most other materials, it may cause less foreign body reaction as an implant.

This was borne out in the late 1940's and by the early 1950's reports appeared in medical journals on the acceptability of silicones as subdermal implants.[51]

One of the earliest of silicone rubber implants was the hydroephalus shunt, dating back to 1955. Originally, the device drained cerebrospinal fluid from the brain and into the blood system via the jugular vein and into the right auricle of the heart. This did create some problems such as blood clotting and infection and revision with a patient's growth. In the 1960's, the Ames Ventriculo-Peritoneal Shunt directed drainage into the peritoneal cavity rather than into the blood stream.[52]

Silicone is a specialty rubber, with outstanding characteristics. Some of these unique properties include resistance to (a) temperature extremes (-50°F to +450°F), (b) weathering, ozone and sunlight, and (c) most dilute acids and alkalis.[53]

The first particle size silica *fumed*, is the major reinforcing filler for developing maximum tensile and tear strength. It is also the major factor for building hardness or durometer. Typical tensile range for medical grade silicones is 1000 to 1400 psi, while tear strength is 100 to 300 pounds per inch of thickness. Shore A durometer can be from 25 to 80, and through blending may be customized to nearly any unit between.

Heat curing silicone rubbers are most commonly vulcanized by using either organic peroxides or a platinum catalyzed system. The latter has no volatile by-products produced during curing and deep sections cure evenly. It produces maximum strength, is reversion resistant, quite clean and a glossy surface.[54]

Room temperature vulcanizing or RTV silicone rubber compounds are vulcanized from either a condensation or addition reaction. The condensation reaction employs a cross-linker and metallic salt catalyst. The addition reaction is achieved via a catalyst such as chloroplatinic acid.

The well-know Medical Adhesive A™ is a one-component RTV silicone rubber where the cross-linker in the material is triggered by atmospheric moisture to produce rubber properties.[55]

The high strength silicone rubbers, vulcanized at higher temperatures fall into two camps. The first, solid rubbers, are processed as is the usual organic rubbers. The second, are the liquid silicone rubbers which have been marketed for the relatively short period of time of about 16 years. Both materials consist of polydimethylsiloxane with reactive vinyl groups, fumed silica reinforcement, and an appropriate cross-linking agent.

Processing methods are different, however, and because of their plastic flowability, the liquid silicones can be pumped to mixers and then to vulcanizing equipment.[56]

Dacron Felt Cuffs: as Anchors and as Infection Barriers

With the first marketed Broviac silicone rubber catheters for parenteral alimentation, an attached Dacron™ cuff was what was used to minimize epidermidis infections.

The Dacron™ material is a felt and generally, after a two or three week period, tissue ingrowth into the cuff results, sealing the tunnel against bacterial invasion form the outside.[57]

The Hickman catheter, also of silicone rubber construction, but larger diameter than the Broviac catheters, again uses Dacron™ polyester felt cuffs. For removal, catheters are simply strongly pulled on and the Dacron™ cuffs usually remain behind, for later removal, if need be.[58]

It is probably wise to mention at this point another cuff material, Vitacuff™. This is a silver impregnated collagen ring placed around the catheter and under the skin at the insertion site. This is, of course, to ward off a catheter-related sepsis and also, collagen does offer additional catheter securement.[59]

Venous Access Port

Regardless of the reservoir material for a venous access disk or port, be it stainless steel, titanium, polysulfone or Delrin™ (polyacetal), the penetrated self-sealing septum is of silicone rubber construction. The material choice for this septum is important since it needs to be non-coring, have good tear and inherent tack for self-sealing.

In spite of a special non-coring needle being used, a Huber-point needle, leaking through coring and fragmenting of the silicone system are quite real possibilities. Besides a top-entry septum, a side-entry approach is also available.

Infectious problems related to chronic access devices are exit-site infections and catheter sepsis. Because exit-site infections are the most common phenomenon, the totally implanted subcutaneous port would offer less of a problem in this respect.[60]

Some of the shortcomings of the subcutaneous port are eliminated with a new implanted port accessed by a catheter-over-needle system, Cath-link™. This item is constructed of implant grade titanium and a stacked internal valve septum of implant grade silicone and an implant grade polyurethane catheter is attached. There is virtually no reservoir for this port.[61]

One of the first totally implanted injection ports was manufactured by the Infusaid[62] Corporation, Sharon, Massachusetts, made available in 1983, and called the Infuse-A-Port and had a titanium chamber and silicone rubber catheter.

Silicone Rubber Cross-Linking Systems

The organic peroxides are the most commonly used vulcanizing agents for the heat cured silicones. A less common method is high energy radiation curing. Obviously, the limiting factor is the high initial cost of the equipment. It does offer the advantage of a tough and reversion resistant rubber.

Newer, millable type of addition reaction rubber compounds were introduced by General Electric in the 1970's. Here the catalyst is a platinum salt at extremely low concentrations. Improvements found with this system are maximum strength, especially for tear resistance, reversion resistance and a less tacky surface, compared to conventional peroxide cross-linking.

Regardless of the cure system, the post curing of silicone rubber parts, especially for biomedical use, should be standard procedure. This step in the process drives off volatile materials, including those chemical by-products of vulcanizations and low molecular weight components, and so reduces the effects that might hinder biocompatibility.

SILICONE RUBBER ATRIAL CATHETERS – COMPARED

Tunneled External CVC's – Silicone Large Bore Catheters

The concept of offering parenteral nutrition through the use of a silicone catheter was conceived in 1970. The experience garnered from use of the silicone rubber atrial catheters with hydrocephalic children suggested such a possibility to Dr. J.W. Broviac.

Dr. J. Broviac's silicone rubber catheter also made use of a Dacron cuff that effectively reduced sepsis associated with other venous catheters. The catheter was brought on stream and marketed in 1973.[63]

A few years later in 1978, Dr. Robert O. Hickman, detailed the rationale for a larger diameter parenteral nutrition catheter. In fact, it is also used for all blood products, infusion of drugs, intravenous solutions and withdrawal of blood. The Hickman catheter was described as having two Dacron felt cuffs, one placed near the venous entrance site and the other at the skin exit site.[64]

Both catheters, cuffed and subcutaneously tunneled contributed to the fantastic advance in increased safety regarding access to central venous circulation for nutritional chemotherapeutic and blood work.[65]

Since 1984, a new, closed system, tip-first inserted, smaller outside diameter catheter, came onto the scene, the Groshong™ catheter. It was a closed distal end with a pressure sensitive two-way valve. The catheter, as for the Hickman and the Broviac catheters, has a Dacron™ cuff and is constructed of silicone rubber. Where the latter two catheters are of a barium sulfate filled silicone for radiopacity, the clear Groshong™ catheter has a barium sulfate filled striping plus a tungsten/liquid silicone tip for added placement visibility.[66]

Silicone rubber is, relatively, a much softer material compared to the stiffer polyurethane (PU), polyethylene or polyvinylchloride central venous catheters.

A study, in vitro, evaluating various materials composition showed the potential of the stiffer materials to do damage to a blood vessel. The silicone catheters and a novel pigtail-ended polyurethane catheter, which has a rounded knuckle rather than a sharp tip at that working end, performed best.[67]

Silicone catheters in animal testing, have shown superiority in reduction of the frequency of central venous thrombosis during total parenteral nutrition (TPN) when compared to polyethylene catheters, (40% versus 20-33%).[68]

The fact that catheter composition is an important factor in thrombogenesis was shown shown in yet another animal study. Significance was attached to the increase of thromboses with rigid catheters. Polyethylene (PE) and Teflon catheters were especially incriminated. Beside PE, TFE-Teflon (polytetrafluoroethylene) catheters, FEP-Teflon (fluorethylene propylene) catheters, silicone catheters and polyurethane catheters were used in these experiments.[69]

If one of the commonly used materials in intravenous catheters could be declared intrinsically resistant to bacterial colonization, it would be enormously important. Alas, such a study in-vitro and in-vivo of Teflon™ (TFE), Silastic™ (Silicone), Vialon™ (segmented polyether PU) and TecoFlex™ (polyether cycloaliphatic PU) show no such relationship.[70]

Thrombogenicity of different central venous catheter materials was the subject of another study. The materials involved were a hydrophilic coated PU, PVC Silicone, Teflon™, and non-coated PU. The least thrombogenic material was determined to be the hydrophilic (Hydromer™) coated PU, followed by the silicone catheter. Surprisingly, the PVC was next and the most thrombogenic catheter was a non-coated PU. In essence, all catheters formed thrombi and fibrin sheaths, but there is a significant difference among the various catheter materials.[71]

PLASTICS – OTHER

Polyethylene

Polyethylene was discovered in 1933 by E.W. Fawcett, R.O. Gibson and with follow up work of M.W. Perrin in 1935, in England. This was the result of high pressure reaction studies.[72]

The first use of a polyethylene (PE) catheter to introduce fluids intravenously was in 1945.[73]

PE is flexible, smooth walled, and without benefit of a plasticizer to produce these qualities. However pure the material may be, studies showed how much more thrombogenic this was compared to silicone rubber.[74]

After the work in 1941 of Dr. P.L. Farima, with a rubber catheter in arteriographic examination, Dr. E.C. Pierce used polyethylene tubing for this procedure in 1951.[75]

Left heart catheterization, using a PE catheter, via a percutaneous transthoracic route, was described in 1958. This procedure was used to determine mitral valve insufficiency, or mitral sterrosis.[76]

PE has been used in balloon angioplasty catheter, both as a balloon material and main catheter shaft as well.

Infusion of cancer chemotherapy through a PE catheter and using percutaneous visceral catheterization, is not a simple process and the infused drug is not efficiently distributed, in addition.[77]

Major problems associated with percutaneous central venous polyethylene catheters are phlebitis and thrombotic in nature.[78]

The case against polyethylene continued with a dog study using polyethylene catheters and Silastic™ catheters. Polyethylene consistently and extensively thrombosed the veins while silicone only showed small thrombus formed at the entry site and was considered minor.[79]

Teflon™

To measure central venous pressures, an over-the-needle Teflon catheter was employed. The passage into the superior vena cava was via the external jugular vein and through use of a flexible angiographic wire catheter guide (J wire).[80]

Nylon™

Right heart catheterization using a tiny bore Nylon™ catheter was briefly described in a letter to Lancet in 1964. The miniature diameter catheters were for severely ill patients and as diagnostic aids.[81]

Nylon was introduced as a fiber material in 1938. Emil Fisher made an analysis of animal protein and W. H. Carothers took this information further, combining amines and acids to make polyamides in long chains, resulting in the production of Nylon. There are over 100 varieties of Nylon. Nylon 6/10 has minimum water absorption. Fillers add to its versatility.[82]

HORIZONS FOR VAD MATERIALS

The need certainly exists for better biocompatible vascular access materials. The question is, can we forecast what will actually transpire form our wish list?

Each human being is unique and what is tolerated by one body may not be the case in another. The best we can hope for is that most, or nearly all, human patients are without an incidence of reaction to a new material. It may not be a total 100% material performance for 100% of the patient's life.

Today, much of research focuses on a few materials for cardiovascular catheters, mainly polyurethanes and silicone as many players. Other materials that will also dominate the vascular implant market will continue to be silicone/polyurethane copolymers and thermoplastic elastomers.

We have seen a steady improvement in the "usual" biomaterials. For instance, PU, where the latest development, producing an ether-free material, has shown in tests to reduce the environment stress cracking (ESC) potential.

For silicone rubber, it too has seen a succession of improvements, in tensile strength, tear strength and less by-products from its platinum catalyst system of curing.

It appears that coatings will be more depended on to help arrive at the near-perfect implant. For example, hydrogel grafting, heparin bonding, albumin/heparin co-bonds, propyl sulfonate, albumin alone, and phospholipid grafting.

These are not new, but what is required of them is improved affinity to the catheter substrates and longer periods of effective viability.

The closer we come to have an implant mimic body tissue, the better the chance for an "implant-friendly" environment.

Besides surface coatings, we can look forward to a succession of future changes in the chemistry of current vascular access materials, additions to a compound such as antioxidants, device design changes, surface changes, as is possible by gas plasma, and through material manufacturing improvements. For example, cleaner, purer materials, filler treatment, better dispersion of ingredients within the silicone compound or polyurethane or other materials should be our concerns. In general, improvements to such basic features as manufacturing practices can always stand a bit more scrutiny.

Development of a material intrinsically resistant to bacterial colonization would be of tremendous importance. To reduce sepsis would be to reduce cost, morbidity and mortality.

Softer materials or novel designs such as pigtails, would allow stiffer materials to be considered for vascular access, if, or course, they offer the much needed improvements in biocompatibility.

We have seen in animal, human, and in-vitro, that certain materials are better than others for bioacceptability. We can capitalize on this information; continue to improve those materials already accepted, though not perfect, and continue to search for better.

It is the demand for an improved quality of life that pushes the biomaterials industry to reduce pain and improve function through major changes in biomaterials device designs and delivery systems. This will be the continuing driving force for the future.

REFERENCES

Allen, P.W., Jones, K.P. (1985). Natural Rubber Science and Technology, pp 1-28.

Babycon, C.R., Barrocas, A., Webb, W.R. (1993). "*A Prospective Randomized Trial Comparing the Silver-Impregnated Collagen Cuff with the Bedside Tunneled Subclavian Catheter.*" Journal of Parenteral and Enteral Nutrition, 17, No. 1, pg 61.

Bard, C.R. (1958). Catalogue #15, p37.

Blitt, C.D., Wright, W.A., Petty, W.C., Webster, T.A. (1974). "*Central Venous Catheterization Via the External Jugular Vein.*" J.A.M.A., 229, No. 7, pg 817.

Borow, M., Crowley, J.G. (1985). "*Evaluation of Central Venous Catheter Thrombogenicity.*" Acta Anaesthesia Scandanavia, 81. pp 59-64.

Bothe, A.J., Daly, J. (1987), "*Technical Aspects of Vascular Access for Infusional Chemotherapy.*" Cancer Chemotherapy by Infusion, pg 67.

Bradley, R.D., Oct. 31, 1964. "*Diagnostic Right Heart Catheterization with Miniature Catheters in Severely Ill Patients.*" The Lancet, pp 941-942.

Broviac, J.W., Cole, J.J., Scriber, B.H. (1973). "*A Silicone Rubber Atrial Catheter for Prolonged Parenteral Alimentation.*" Surgery, Gynecology and Obstetrics, pp 136, 602, 603.

Brookman, R.S. (1991). A New PVC Based Polymer for Medical Applications. 1991 Antec (SPE) MPD Program Abstracts.

Camp, L.D. (1988). "Care *of the Groshong Catheter.*" Oncology Nursing Forum, 15, No.6, pg 745.

Davis, H. (1976). *"Preface of Her Translation of Werner Forssman's Autobiography."* Experiment on Myself, Memoirs of a Surgeon in Germany. IX.

DiCostanzo, J., Sastre, B., Choux, R., Reynier, J.P., Noirclerc, M., Cano, N., and Martin, J. (1984). *"Experimental Approach to Prevention of Catheter-Related Central Venous Thrombosis."* Journal of Parenteral and Enteral Nutrition, 8, No. 3, pp 293-297.

DiConstanzo, J., Sastre, B., Choux, R., Kasparian, M. (1988). "Mechanism of Thrombogenesis during Total Parenteral Nutrition: Role of Catheter Composition." Journal of Parenteral and Enteral Nutrition, 12, No. 2, pp 190-193.

DuBois, J. H. (1967). Plastics, pg 47, pg 54.

DuBois, J.H., John, F.W. (1967). Plastics, pg 12.

Ensminger, W.D., Walker, S.C., Knul, J.A., Andrews, J.C. (1993). "Initial Clinical Evaluation of a New Implanted Port Accessed by Catheter-Over-Needle System." Journal of Infusional Chemotherapy, pg 200.

Farinas, P. L. (1941). "New Techniques for Arterio-Graphic Examination of Abdominal Aorta and Its Branches." American Journal of Roetgenology. 46, pg 641.

Fisher, P.L. (1957). "Chemistry of Natural and Synthetic Rubbers." Chapter 9. Synthetic Rubbers. Pg 133.

Gilsdorf, J.R., Wilson, K., Beals, T.F. (1989). "Bacterial Colonization of Intravenous Catheter Materials In Vitro and In Vivo." Surgery, 106, pp 37-44.

Golomb, F.M., Sammons, B.P., and Wright, J.C. (April 20, 1964), "Percutaneous Visceral Catheterization for Infusion Cancer Chemotherapy." J.A.M.A., Vol. 188, No.3, pp 225.

Gravenstein, N., Blockshear, R.H. (1991). "In Vitro Evaluation of Relative Perforating Potential of Central Venous Catheter: Comparison of Materials, Selected Models, Number of Lumens, and Angle of Incidence to Simulated Membrane." Journal of Clinical Monitoring, 7, No. 1, pp 1-6.

Greene, F. L., Moore, W., Strickland, G., McFarland, J. (1988). "Comparison of a Totally Implantable Access Device for Chemotherapy (Port-A-Cath) and Long-Term Percutaneous Catheterization (Brovia)." Southern Medical Journal, 81, No.5, pg 581.

Hickman, R.O., Buckner, C.D., Clift, R.A., Sanders, J.E., Stewart, P., and, Thomas, E.D. (1979). "A Modified Right Atrial Catheter for Access to the Venous System in Marrow Transplant Recipients." Surgery, Gynecology and Obstetrics, 148, pp 871-873.

Journal of American Medical Association (J.A.M.A.) (1851). "Minutes of the 4th Annual Meeting, Charlestown, South Carolina." Catheter Extemporaneous, pg 265.

J.A.M.A. (1881). "Minutes of 32nd Annual Meeting Richmond, Virginia." New Catheters, Tuesday May 3, 1881.

J.A.M.A. (1884). III, No. 1, pg 157.

J.A.M.A. (Jan. 11, 1930). Klinische Wochenschrift, Berlin, (Nov 5 1929), W. Forssman, 94, No. 2, 143, pg 2085.

J.A.M.A. (12/20/41). 117, No. 25, pg 2173.

J.A.M.A. (1955). 158, No. 17, pg 1498.

J.A.M.A. (December 15, 1956). 162, No. 13, pg 1492.

J.A.M.A. (7/26/1958). 167, No. 13, pp 1606 and 1611.

J.A.M.A. (9/19/1959). Indwelling Catheters (Gristch and Ballenger), 171, No. 3, pp 125 and 285.

J.A.M.A. (5/13/1968). 204, No. 7, pg 118.

J.A.M.A. (1973). Transfemoral Pacing with Balloon-Tipped Catheters. Meister, S.G., Banks, U.S., Hellfant, R.H., 225, No. 7, pg 712.

J.A.M.A. (1973). Medical News. 226, No. 8, pg 843.

J.A.M.A. (1975). 233, No. 8, pg 865.

Jeckel, N.C. (1967), U.S. Patent 3,336,918, *"Radiopaque, Urethane-Coated Catheter and Method of Coating Same."*

Kambic, H.E., Nose, Y. (1991). Blood Compatible Materials and Devices. Chapter 8, pp 141-143.

Lancet (1830). pp 778-779.

Lancet (April 13, 1946). pg 541.

Lancet (September 7, 1957). Professor A. Montanari, pg 480.

Lancet (September, 28, 1957). pg 643.

Lower, R. (1669). Tractus de Corde, Early Science in Oxford London, Oxford Press, 9, pg 1932.

Lynch, W. (1978). Handbook of Silicone Fabrication. 36. pg 147.

McMillan, C.R. (1945). *"Elastomers for Biomedical Applications."* Rubber Chemistry and Technology, July-August 1994, 67, No. 3, pp 429-430.

Meyers, L. (1945). *"Intravenous Catheterization."* American Journal of Nursing, 45, pp 930-931.

Morton, M., Montermoso, J.C. (1962). *"Silicone Rubbers."* Introduction to Rubber Technology. 16, pg 384.

Niederhuber, J.E., Ensminger, W., Gyves, J.W. Liepman, M., Doan, K., Cozzi, E. (1982). *"Totally Implanted Venous and Arterial Access System to Replace External Catheters in Cancer Treatment."* Surgery, pg 706.

Noble, M.G. (1978). *"Silicone Elastomers."* The Vanderbilt Rubber Handbook. pg 224.

Pasquariello, C.A., Lowe, D.A. (1993). Pediatrics, 91, pg 983.

Poly Medics Industries (1994). Chrono Flex™ Biostable Polyurethane Elastomers. pg 5.

Robinson, C.N. (1949). Meet the Plastics. pg 13.

Ryu, G., Han, D., Kim, Y., and Min, B. (1992). ASAIO Transactions. 38 (3), M644.

Sarewitz, A.B., Muehsam, G.E., Baker, S.J. (1958). Left Heart Catheterization. 55, No. 9, pp 468-470.

Sharma, C.P., Szycher, M. (1991). Blood Compatible Materials and Devices. Technomic Publishing Co., Lancaster PA, pg 35.

Swan, H.J.C., Ganz, W., Forrester, J., et al. (1970). *"Catheterization of the Heart is Man with Use of a Flow-Directed Balloon-Tipped Catheter."* New England Journal of Medicine. 283, pp 447-451.

Szycher, M. (1992). *"Seminar: Advances in Medical Plastics"*, April 21-24, 1992, Boston, MA 14.2

Szycher, M., Siciliano, A.A., Reed, A.M. (1991). *"Polyurethanes in Medical Devices."* Medical Design and Material.

Szycher, M., Reed, A.M., (1992). *"Biostable Polyurethane Elastomers."* Medical Device Technology.

Taylor, D. (1989). *"Percutaneous (Non-Tunneled) Central Lines."* Bavan Conference

Walker, S., Calzone, K. (1994). Navan, 1 No. 2, pg 7.

Walters, M.B., Stanger, H.A.D., Rotem, C.E. (1972). *"Complications with Percutaneous Central Venous Catheters."* J.A.M.A. 220, No. 11, pg 1455.

Welch, G.W., McKeel Jr, D.W., Silverstein, P. and Walker, H.L. (1974). *"The Role of Catheter Composition in the Development of Thrombophlebitis."* Surgery, Gynecology & Obstetrics, 138, pp 421-424.

Wilbur MD, C.K. (1979). Antique Medical Instruments, pg 74.

Wrobel, D. (1991). *"Structure and Properties of Hot-Vulcanized Silicone Rubbers."* Silicone Chemistry and Technology, pg 61.

NOTES

1. Wilbur, 1979
2. Wilbur, 1979
3. Wilbur 1979
4. Journal of American Medical Association, 1884
5. American Medical Association, 1851
6. Lancet, 1830
7. American Medical Association, 1881
8. Journal of American Medical Association, 1884
9. Lower, 1669
10. Taylor, 1989
11. Davies, 1976
12. Lancet, 1957
13. Lancet, 1957
14. Davies, 1976
15. JAMA 1956
16. Lancet, 1957
17. JAMA, 1930
18. Farinas, 1941
19. Lancet, 1946
20. JAMA 1930
21. JANA 1956
22. Pasquariello & Lowe, 1993
23. Allen & Jones, 1985
24. Allen & Jones 1985
25. Sharma & Szycher, 1991
26. Szycher, 1992
27. McMillin, 1994

28 Kambic, H.E. & Nose, Y., 1991
29 Ryu et all, 1992
30 Szycher et al, 1991
31 Szycher, Reed, 1992
32 Szycher, Reed 1992
33 Poly Medica Industries, 1994
34 Jeckel, 1967
35 *JAMA*, 12/20/41
36 Walker & Calzone, 1994
37 *JAMA*, 9/19/59
38 Curelaru et al, 1984
39 *JAMA*, 1959
40 *JAMA*, 1969
41 *JAMA*, 1973
42 *JAMA*, 1973
43 Swan, H.J.C. et al, 1970
44 *JAMA*, 1975
45 Taylor, 1989
46 Brookman, 1991
47 Dubois & John, 1967
48 Robinson, 1949
49 Braley, 1974
50 Fisher, 1957
51 Dow Corning Corporation, 1973
52 Dow Corning Corporation, 1973
53 Morton, et al, 1962
54 Lynch, 1978
55 Noble, 1978
56 Wrobel, 1991
57 Broviac, et al, 1973
58 Hickman, et al, 1979
59 Babycos, et al, 1993
60 Bothe, et al, 1987
61 Ensminger, 1993
62 Niederhuber, et al, 1982
63 Broviac, et al, 1973
64 Hickman, et al, 1979
65 Green, et al, 1988

[66] Camp, 1988
[67] Gravenstein, et al, 1991
[68] DiCostanzo, et al, 1984
[69] DiCostanzo, et al, 1988
[70] Gilsdorf, et al, 1989
[71] Borow, et al, 1985
[72] Dubois, 1967
[73] Meyers, 1945
[74] *JAMA*, 7/26/58
[75] *JAMA*, 1955
[76] Sarewitz, et al, 1958
[77] Galomb, et al, 1964
[78] Walters, et al, 1972
[79] Welch, et al, 1974
[80] Blithe, et al, 1974
[81] Bradley, 1964
[82] DuBois, 1967

www.ingramcontent.com/pod-product-compliance
Lightning Source LLC
Chambersburg PA
CBHW021049180526
45163CB00005B/2358